CODY SMITH

100 Pull-Ups a Day 30 Day Challenge

Gain Muscle, Massive Strength, and Increase Your Pull up, Chin up Rep Count Using This One Killer Exercise Program | at Home Workouts | No Gym Required |

First published by Nelaco Press 2021

Copyright © 2021 by Cody Smith

The exercises provided by the author (and the publisher) are for educational and entertainment purposes only, and are not to be interpreted as a recommendation for a specific course of action. Exercise is not without its risks, and this or any other exercise program may result in injury. They include but are not limited to: risk of injury, aggravation of a pre-existing condition, or adverse effect of over-exertion such as muscle strain, abnormal blood pressure, fainting, disorders of heartbeat, and very rare instances of heart attack. To reduce the risk of injury, before beginning this or any exercise program, please consult a healthcare provider for appropriate exercise prescription and safety precautions. The exercises instructions and advice presented are in no way intended as a substitute for medical consultation. The author (and the publisher) disclaims any liability from and in connection with this program. As with any exercise program, if at any point during your workout you begin to feel faint, dizzy, or have physical discomfort, you should stop immediately and consult a physician.

First edition

ISBN: 978-1-952381-06-5

This book was professionally typeset on Reedsy.
Find out more at reedsy.com

Contents

Before You Begin

Hey reader, thanks for grabbing a copy of the book.

If you are looking to pair this workout program with a complimentary guide to shed weight and boost your growth hormones to build more muscle faster, then I've got you covered.

Seems crazy to do both at the same time, but you can.

Better still, it is stupid easy.

Oh, and it is free. You can do this method anytime you want, anywhere for the rest of your life.

I usually sell this information, but I want you to have it.

You can get a copy from your cell phone from a simple text.

Seriously, get your phone out and text BOOST to (678) 506-7543.

Cheers!

Introduction: How to Use This Book

Let me be the first to welcome you to the 100 pull-ups a day 30 day challenge program.

The next 30 days are going to be awesome as you work your way to completing literally 3000 pull-ups.

That's more than most people do in a lifetime.

I'm a little obsessed with pull-ups because they are such a killer exercise, a show of strength, and a phenomenal way to workout with just your body and a bar.

Speaking of bars, you'll need a pull-up bar to begin this program.

Make sure the one you use is safe and secure.

For the love of bacon and pineapple pizza, don't use sketchy pull-ups bars like tree branches, a shower curtain rod, or the family chandelier.

You're just asking to injure yourself, goober.

This program starts with an initial pull-up assessment to determine where you need to start in the program.

Don't skip the assessment.

Once you complete the assessment, your 30 day challenge will start the very next day with whatever workout you're assigned from the post-assessment results.

While you're starting out in the program, you'll most likely be very sore early on in the program. Your body has not adapted to completing 100 pull-ups a day yet. That's okay, if the soreness is bearable, you can continue with the program.

If the soreness is unbearable, take a break for a few days until you recover and hop right back into the program where you left off.

You will also experience blisters, which I like to call bar bubbles, along the way. This is normal. Treat them and move on. If the blisters make it unreasonable to continue, let them heal and come back where you left off.

If you can't complete your workout one day or have to skip a day here and there, don't fret. That's 100% okay and won't throw you way off. Quitting is the only no-no.

Remember, this is a challenge. It's supposed to be challenging.

If it's a cakewalk, you've gained nothing but wasted time.

This brings me to the most important question:

Are you ready to accept the challenge?

Of course, you are!

You may not feel 100% ready but you've 100% accepted this challenge.

You will be victorious no matter how hard it gets.

With that said, welcome to the 100 pull-ups a day challenge.

Head to the initial pull-up assessment and let the games begin.

Initial Pull-up Assessment

Welcome to the initial pull-up assessment portion of this program. This is where you're going to check your current repetition count to see how many pull-ups you can actually perform without stopping.

This number will determine which workout you need to start with as you make your way through the 100 pull-up challenge program.

As you can imagine, you'll need a pull-up bar to complete your assessment so go ahead and find one handy to get started.

Make sure you are doing full pull-ups going all the way through the motion palms facing away from you. Starting at the bottom with arms straight and shoulders engaged, pull up to the bar so your chin goes over the bar. Then descend back down in a controlled manner to the start position.

Alright, you should be near a pull-up bar. Go ahead complete as many pull-ups as you can without stopping.

When you're done, make a note of how many you completed and head to the post assessment results section.

Post Assessment Results

Welcome to the post assessment results section.

This is where you'll see what workout you'll start with based on the number of pull-ups you completed during the assessment.

Still got that number in your head?

Good.

- If you completed <6 pull-ups, your first workout starting tomorrow will be Workout 1.
- If you completed between 6 - 7 pull-ups, your first workout will be Workout 2.
- If you completed between 8 - 9 pull-ups, your first workout will be Workout 3.
- If you completed 10 pull-ups, your first workout will be Workout 4.
- If you completed between 11 - 12 pull-ups, your first workout will be Workout 5.
- If you completed between 13 - 14 pull-ups, your first workout will be Workout 6.
- If you completed 15 pull-ups, your first workout will be Workout 7.
- If you completed between 16 - 17 pull-ups, your first workout will be

Workout 8.
- If you completed between 18 - 19 pull-ups, your first workout will be Workout 9.
- If you completed 20 pull-ups, your first workout will be Workout 10.
- If you completed between 21 - 22 pull-ups, your first workout will be Workout 11.
- If you completed between 23 - 24 pull-ups, your first workout will be Workout 12.
- If you completed 25 pull-ups, your first workout will be Workout 13.
- If you completed between 26 - 27 pull-ups, your first workout will be Workout 14.
- If you completed between 28 - 29 pull-ups, your first workout will be Workout 15.
- If you completed 30 or more pull-ups, your first workout will be Workout 16.

Don't fret if you didn't complete a lot of pull-ups. The point of the challenge is to start where you are and complete the full 30 days of 100 pull-ups a day. Not to be some amazing pull-up champion on day 1.

With that said, you know where you need to start starting tomorrow with your very first 100 pull-ups a day workout.

See you there.

Completed Workouts Checklist

Check these off as you complete them:

_____Workout 1

_____Workout 2

_____Workout 3

_____Workout 4

_____Workout 5

_____Workout 6

_____Workout 7

_____Workout 8

_____Workout 9

_____Workout 10

_____Workout 11

_____Workout 12

_____Workout 13

_____Workout 14

_____Workout 15

_____Workout 16

30 Day Completion Checklist

Date started: _____ (DD/MM/YYYY)

_____Day 1

_____Day 2

_____Day 3

_____Day 4

_____Day 5

_____Day 6

_____Day 7

_____Day 8

_____Day 9

_____Day 10

_____Day 11

_____Day 12

_____Day 13

_____Day 14

_____Day 15

_____Day 16

_____Day 17

_____Day 18

_____Day 19

_____Day 20

_____Day 21

_____Day 22

_____Day 23

_____Day 24
_____Day 25
_____Day 26
_____Day 27
_____Day 28
_____Day 29
_____Day 30

Pre and Post Challenge Measurements

The following measurements are 100% optional and are not required to start or finish the program. I know some people will be curious to know other areas that are positively affected by completing the challenge.

Starting weight: _____

Starting pull-up rep max: _____

Starting body row rep max: _____

Starting standing row max: _____

Starting cable pull down max: _____

Starting bicep measurement: _____

Ending weight: _____

Ending pull-up rep max: _____

Ending body row rep max: _____

Ending standing row max: _____

Ending cable pull down max: _____

Ending bicep measurement: _____

Workout 1

Welcome to Workout 1 of the 100 pull-ups a day 30 day challenge.

For this workout, 1 pull-up is performed every minute.

Because this is such a long workout, do your best to at least complete 50 pull-ups. Once you get stronger, re-do the initial assessment to work your way up the workout chain where the workouts are harder but take less time to complete.

This workout is way easier with an interval timer app. I suggest downloading one onto your phone with the following settings for this workout:

Intervals: 100

Time per interval: 1:03

That time will give you enough time to complete the number of correct pull-ups and enough time to rest between sets. The interval app also makes it easy to determine what set you're on.

With that said, go ahead and get started.

Come back in when you are done.

* * *

Way to go!

You completed 100 pull-ups today!

That's more than most people do in a year.

If that workout was too easy, consider moving up to the next workout.

If that workout was still fairly challenging, continue with this workout tomorrow.

That's all I've got for you today. See you tomorrow, champ!

Workout 2

Welcome to Workout 2 of the 100 pull-ups a day 30 day challenge.

For this workout, 1 or 2 pull-ups are performed every minute.

The first 25 sets are 2 pull-ups each.

The last 50 sets are 1 pull-up each.

Because this is such a long workout, do your best to at least complete 50 pull-ups. Once you get stronger, re-do the initial assessment to work your way up the workout chain where the workouts are harder but take less time to complete.

This workout is way easier with an interval timer app. I suggest downloading one onto your phone with the following settings for this workout:

Intervals: 75

Time per interval: 1:06

That time will give you enough time to complete the number of correct pull-ups and enough time to rest between sets. The interval app also makes it easy to determine what set you're on.

With that said, go ahead and get started.

Come back in when you are done.

* * *

Way to go!

You completed 100 pull-ups today!

That's more than most people do in a year.

If that workout was too easy, consider moving up to the next workout.

If that workout was still fairly challenging, continue with this workout tomorrow.

That's all I've got for you today. See you tomorrow, champ!

Workout 3

Welcome to Workout 3 of the 100 pull-ups a day 30 day challenge.

For this workout, 1 or 2 pull-ups are performed every minute.

The first 40 sets are 2 pull-ups each.

The last 20 sets are 1 pull-up each.

Because this is such a long workout, do your best to at least complete 50 pull-ups. Once you get stronger, re-do the initial assessment to work your way up the workout chain where the workouts are harder but take less time to complete.

This workout is way easier with an interval timer app. I suggest downloading one onto your phone with the following settings for this workout:

Intervals: 60

Time per interval: 1:06

That time will give you enough time to complete the number of correct pull-ups and enough time to rest between sets. The interval app also makes it easy to determine what set you're on.

With that said, go ahead and get started.

Come back in when you are done.

* * *

Way to go!

You completed 100 pull-ups today!

That's more than most people do in a year.

If that workout was too easy, consider moving up to the next workout.

If that workout was still fairly challenging, continue with this workout tomorrow.

That's all I've got for you today. See you tomorrow, champ!

Workout 4

Welcome to Workout 1 of the 100 pull-ups a day 30 day challenge.

For this workout, 2 pull-ups are performed every minute.

Because this is such a long workout, do your best to at least complete 50 pull-ups. Once you get stronger, re-do the initial assessment to work your way up the workout chain where the workouts are harder but take less time to complete.

This workout is way easier with an interval timer app. I suggest downloading one onto your phone with the following settings for this workout:

Intervals: 50

Time per interval: 1:06

That time will give you enough time to complete the number of correct pull-ups and enough time to rest between sets. The interval app also makes it easy to determine what set you're on.

With that said, go ahead and get started.

Come back in when you are done.

* * *

Way to go!

You completed 100 pull-ups today!

That's more than most people do in a year.

If that workout was too easy, consider moving up to the next workout.

If that workout was still fairly challenging, continue with this workout tomorrow.

That's all I've got for you today. See you tomorrow, champ!

Workout 5

Welcome to Workout 5 of the 100 pull-ups a day 30 day challenge.

For this workout, 2 or 3 pull-ups are performed every minute.

The first 14 sets are 3 pull-ups each.

The last 29 sets are 2 pull-ups each.

This workout is way easier with an interval timer app. I suggest downloading one onto your phone with the following settings for this workout:

Intervals: 43

Time per interval: 1:09

That time will give you enough time to complete the number of correct pull-ups and enough time to rest between sets. The interval app also makes it easy to determine what set you're on.

With that said, go ahead and get started.

Come back in when you are done.

* * *

Way to go!

You completed 100 pull-ups today!

That's more than most people do in a year.

If that workout was too easy, consider moving up to the next workout.

If that workout was still fairly challenging, continue with this workout tomorrow.

That's all I've got for you today. See you tomorrow, champ!

Workout 6

Welcome to Workout 6 of the 100 pull-ups a day 30 day challenge.

For this workout, 2 or 3 pull-ups are performed every minute.

The first 24 sets are 3 pull-ups each.

The last 14 sets are 2 pull-ups each.

This workout is way easier with an interval timer app. I suggest downloading one onto your phone with the following settings for this workout:

Intervals: 38

Time per interval: 1:09

That time will give you enough time to complete the number of correct pull-ups and enough time to rest between sets. The interval app also makes it easy to determine what set you're on.

With that said, go ahead and get started.

Come back in when you are done.

* * *

Way to go!

You completed 100 pull-ups today!

That's more than most people do in a year.

If that workout was too easy, consider moving up to the next workout.

If that workout was still fairly challenging, continue with this workout tomorrow.

That's all I've got for you today. See you tomorrow, champ!

Workout 7

Welcome to Workout 7 of the 100 pull-ups a day 30 day challenge.

For this workout, 3 pull-ups are performed every minute.

The first 33 sets are 3 pull-ups each.

The last set is 1 pull-up.

This workout is way easier with an interval timer app. I suggest downloading one onto your phone with the following settings for this workout:

Intervals: 34

Time per interval: 1:09

That time will give you enough time to complete the number of correct pull-ups and enough time to rest between sets. The interval app also makes it easy to determine what set you're on.

With that said, go ahead and get started.

Come back in when you are done.

* * *

Way to go!

You completed 100 pull-ups today!

That's more than most people do in a year.

If that workout was too easy, consider moving up to the next workout.

If that workout was still fairly challenging, continue with this workout tomorrow.

That's all I've got for you today. See you tomorrow, champ!

Workout 8

Welcome to Workout 8 of the 100 pull-ups a day 30 day challenge.

For this workout, 3 or 4 pull-ups are performed every minute.

The first 10 sets are 4 pull-ups each.

The last 20 sets are 3 pull-ups each.

This workout is way easier with an interval timer app. I suggest downloading one onto your phone with the following settings for this workout:

Intervals: 30

Time per interval: 1:12

That time will give you enough time to complete the number of correct pull-ups and enough time to rest between sets. The interval app also makes it easy to determine what set you're on.

With that said, go ahead and get started.

Come back in when you are done.

* * *

Way to go!

You completed 100 pull-ups today!

That's more than most people do in a year.

If that workout was too easy, consider moving up to the next workout.

If that workout was still fairly challenging, continue with this workout tomorrow.

That's all I've got for you today. See you tomorrow, champ!

Workout 9

Welcome to Workout 9 of the 100 pull-ups a day 30 day challenge.

For this workout, 3 or 4 pull-ups are performed every minute.

The first 18 sets are 4 pull-ups each.

The next 9 sets are 3 pull-ups each.

The last set is 1 pull-up.

This workout is way easier with an interval timer app. I suggest downloading one onto your phone with the following settings for this workout:

Intervals: 28

Time per interval: 1:12

That time will give you enough time to complete the number of correct pull-ups and enough time to rest between sets. The interval app also makes it easy to determine what set you're on.

With that said, go ahead and get started.

Come back in when you are done.

* * *

Way to go!

You completed 100 pull-ups today!

That's more than most people do in a year.

If that workout was too easy, consider moving up to the next workout.

If that workout was still fairly challenging, continue with this workout tomorrow.

That's all I've got for you today. See you tomorrow, champ!

Workout 10

Welcome to Workout 10 of the 100 pull-ups a day 30 day challenge.

For this workout, 4 pull-ups are performed every minute.

This workout is way easier with an interval timer app. I suggest downloading one onto your phone with the following settings for this workout:

Intervals: 25

Time per interval: 1:12

That time will give you enough time to complete the number of correct pull-ups and enough time to rest between sets. The interval app also makes it easy to determine what set you're on.

With that said, go ahead and get started.

Come back in when you are done.

* * *

Way to go!

You completed 100 pull-ups today!

That's more than most people do in a year.

If that workout was too easy, consider moving up to the next workout.

If that workout was still fairly challenging, continue with this workout tomorrow.

That's all I've got for you today. See you tomorrow, champ!

Workout 11

Welcome to Workout 11 of the 100 pull-ups a day 30 day challenge.

For this workout, 4 or 5 pull-ups are performed every minute.

The first 8 sets are 5 pull-ups each.

The last 15 sets are 4 pull-ups each.

This workout is way easier with an interval timer app. I suggest downloading one onto your phone with the following settings for this workout:

Intervals: 23

Time per interval: 1:15

That time will give you enough time to complete the number of correct pull-ups and enough time to rest between sets. The interval app also makes it easy to determine what set you're on.

With that said, go ahead and get started.

Come back in when you are done.

* * *

Way to go!

You completed 100 pull-ups today!

That's more than most people do in a year.

If that workout was too easy, consider moving up to the next workout.

If that workout was still fairly challenging, continue with this workout tomorrow.

That's all I've got for you today. See you tomorrow, champ!

Workout 12

Welcome to Workout 12 of the 100 pull-ups a day 30 day challenge.

For this workout, 4 or 5 pull-ups are performed every minute.

The first 14 sets are 5 pull-ups each.

The next 7 sets are 4 pull-ups each.

The last set is 2 pull-ups.

This workout is way easier with an interval timer app. I suggest downloading one onto your phone with the following settings for this workout:

Intervals: 22

Time per interval: 1:15

That time will give you enough time to complete the number of correct pull-ups and enough time to rest between sets. The interval app also makes it easy to determine what set you're on.

With that said, go ahead and get started.

Come back in when you are done.

* * *

Way to go!

You completed 100 pull-ups today!

That's more than most people do in a year.

If that workout was too easy, consider moving up to the next workout.

If that workout was still fairly challenging, continue with this workout tomorrow.

That's all I've got for you today. See you tomorrow, champ!

Workout 13

Welcome to Workout 13 of the 100 pull-ups a day 30 day challenge.

For this workout, 5 pull-ups are performed every minute.

This workout is way easier with an interval timer app. I suggest downloading one onto your phone with the following settings for this workout:

Intervals: 20

Time per interval: 1:15

That time will give you enough time to complete the number of correct pull-ups and enough time to rest between sets. The interval app also makes it easy to determine what set you're on.

With that said, go ahead and get started.

Come back in when you are done.

* * *

Way to go!

You completed 100 pull-ups today!

That's more than most people do in a year.

If that workout was too easy, consider moving up to the next workout.

If that workout was still fairly challenging, continue with this workout tomorrow.

That's all I've got for you today. See you tomorrow, champ!

Workout 14

Welcome to Workout 14 of the 100 pull-ups a day 30 day challenge.

For this workout, 5 or 6 pull-ups are performed every minute.

The first 6 sets are 6 pull-ups each.

The next 12 sets are 5 pull-ups each.

The last set is 4 pull-ups.

This workout is way easier with an interval timer app. I suggest downloading one onto your phone with the following settings for this workout:

Intervals: 19

Time per interval: 1:18

That time will give you enough time to complete the number of correct pull-ups and enough time to rest between sets. The interval app also makes it easy to determine what set you're on.

With that said, go ahead and get started.

Come back in when you are done.

* * *

Way to go!

You completed 100 pull-ups today!

That's more than most people do in a year.

If that workout was too easy, consider moving up to the next workout.

If that workout was still fairly challenging, continue with this workout tomorrow.

That's all I've got for you today. See you tomorrow, champ!

Workout 15

Welcome to Workout 15 of the 100 pull-ups a day 30 day challenge.

For this workout, 5 or 6 pull-ups are performed every minute.

The first 11 sets are 6 pull-ups each.

The next 6 sets are 5 pull-ups each.

The last set is 4 pull-ups.

This workout is way easier with an interval timer app. I suggest downloading one onto your phone with the following settings for this workout:

Intervals: 18

Time per interval: 1:18

That time will give you enough time to complete the number of correct pull-ups and enough time to rest between sets. The interval app also makes it easy to determine what set you're on.

With that said, go ahead and get started.

Come back in when you are done.

* * *

Way to go!

You completed 100 pull-ups today!

That's more than most people do in a year.

If that workout was too easy, consider moving up to the next workout.

If that workout was still fairly challenging, continue with this workout tomorrow.

That's all I've got for you today. See you tomorrow, champ!

Workout 16

Welcome to Workout 16 of the 100 pull-ups a day 30 day challenge.

For this workout, 6 pull-ups are performed every minute.

The first 16 sets are 6 pull-ups each.

The last set is 4 pull-ups.

This workout is way easier with an interval timer app. I suggest downloading one onto your phone with the following settings for this workout:

Intervals: 17

Time per interval: 1:18

That time will give you enough time to complete the number of correct pull-ups and enough time to rest between sets. The interval app also makes it easy to determine what set you're on.

With that said, go ahead and get started.

Come back in when you are done.

* * *

Way to go!

You completed 100 pull-ups today!

That's more than most people do in a year.

That's all I've got for you today. See you tomorrow, champ!

Post 30 Day Assessment

Hey champ, before we get into the post-assessment, I'd like to ask you for a quick favor.

I'm going to be greedy for a minute here and ask you to leave a review for the book.

Maybe give a star for every blister or callous you got from this program.

Reviews are a pain to get but it'll only take a minute or two to leave one.

So while you're warming up to destroy this assessment, pull your phone out and scan this QR code:

It'll take you straight to the book's page on Amazon.

Scroll to the bottom and click 'Leave a Customer Review.' Leave a star rating, say a few words, and click submit.

It's that simple!

Once you're done, come back to crush your assessment.

* * *

You accepted the 30 day challenge, you completed the 30 day challenge, and now it's time to see where you are now after nailing down 3000 pull-ups.

This is pretty exciting.

All that hard work, dedication, and blisters to get to this point.

I hope to goodness sake you've allowed a couple days to recover between the 30th day of your challenge and now.

You'll see much better results that way.

With that said, get ready to crush this assessment.

Remember that number you started out with during the first assessment?

Go ahead and say that number out loud.

You're about to blow past that number.

Go ahead complete as many pull-ups as you can without stopping.

* * *

How'd you do?

Satisfied with your new number?

Yes and no right?

Yes because you knocked out way more reps and no because you're hungry for more!

Don't be afraid to take a week off and start the challenge again with your new assessment number.

Conclusion

Hey champ, I really hope you enjoyed the 100 pull-ups a day 30 day program.

I hope it was challenging, I hope you pushed yourself, and I hope your post-assessment was worthy of a killer high five.

If you're thirsty for more challenges, we've got more where this came from.

And if you've enjoyed this book, do take a second to leave a review.

Those jokers are hard to get but will only take a minute or two for you to leave one.

Until next time, champ.